Healthy Eating Routine to Balance Hormone

Heal your metabolism and shed up to 4 pounds a day

Dr. Robert R. Dixon

Healthy eating routine to balance hormone

Copyright © Dr. Robert R. Dixon, 2023

The information in this book is presented purely from the author's experience and passed on for educational and informational purposes. While every effort has been made to provide accurate and up-to-date information, the author and publisher make no warranties or representations concerning the accuracy, applicability, or completeness of the content.

Dr. Robert. R. Dixon

Healthy eating routine to balance hormone

2

Dr. Robert. R. Dixon

Healthy eating routine to balance hormone

Table of content

Dr. Robert. R. Dixon

Healthy eating routine to balance hormone

Dr. Robert. R. Dixon

Dr. Robert. R. Dixon

INTRODUCTION

People frequently battle with weight control, sluggish metabolisms, and hormone imbalances in today's fast-paced and stressful society. Adopting a healthy eating regimen is a solution that not only solves these issues but also enhances general well-being. You can reset your hormones, speed up your metabolism, and lose up to 4 pounds a day by giving your body the right nutrition and making conscious decisions. This post will discuss the value of maintaining a nutritious diet, how it affects hormones and metabolism, and practical methods for assisting you in reaching your weight

Dr. Robert. R. Dixon

Healthy eating routine to balance hormone

loss objectives. Now let's get started and learn how eating a balanced, nutrient-dense diet may change your life.

Dr. Robert. R. Dixon

CHAPTER 1:

KNOWLEDGE OF METABOLISM AND HORMONE

1.1 Hormones' Function in Our Bodies

Chemical messengers called hormones are essential for controlling several bodily processes. They are released by glands and reach their intended organs via circulation, where they attach to receptors and cause certain reactions. The preservation of homeostasis, or the equilibrium of the body's internal systems, is one of the key roles of hormones. For instance, by directing cells to take up glucose from the blood, the hormone insulin helps control blood sugar levels. Hormones are also essential for development and growth. Hormones like estrogen and testosterone are in charge of bodily changes like growth spurts and the emergence of traits specific to secondary sex throughout puberty. Hormones also control mood, energy levels, and metabolism. For example, when the body experiences stress, the hormone cortisol is released, which aids in overcoming both emotional and physical obstacles. While the roles of the many hormones vary, they all cooperate to keep our bodies operating as they

Dr. Robert. R. Dixon

should. A hormone imbalance can result in several different health issues. Consequently, it's critical to lead a healthy lifestyle and get medical attention if hormonal imbalances are thought to be present.

1.2 The Impact of Metabolism on Weight Loss

The intricate metabolic reactions that take place inside the body to transform food into energy are referred to as metabolism. It is essential to managing weight and general health. The impact of metabolism on weight loss is one of the main reasons why many people struggle with losing weight. Since metabolism controls how many calories the body needs to burn to operate, it is important

Dr. Robert. R. Dixon

for weight loss. The body burns more calories and weight loss is easier the faster the metabolism. Conversely, a slower metabolism results in fewer calories being expended, which makes weight loss more difficult. A person's metabolism is influenced by several variables, such as age, gender, heredity, food preferences, and degree of physical activity. Our metabolism slows down as we get older, which makes it harder to lose weight. Because they often have more muscle mass than women, men often have a faster metabolism. Because certain people are born with a naturally faster or slower metabolism, our genetics also play a part. Weight loss and metabolism can also be impacted by dietary practices. Consuming a diet rich in macronutrients (carbohydrates, proteins, and fats) and well-balanced will help increase metabolism and promote weight loss. However, crash dieting or extreme calorie restriction might slow down metabolism, which makes weight loss more difficult. Increasing physical exercise is also essential for increasing metabolism. Frequent physical activity, particularly strength training, can boost muscle mass, which raises metabolism. This indicates that people with higher muscle mass burn more calories than people with lower muscle mass, even when they are at rest. In general, establishing a calorie deficit—that is, taking fewer

Dr. Robert. R. Dixon

calories than the body expels—is the key to harnessing metabolism to support weight loss. People can lose weight more successfully if they combine regular physical activity with a balanced diet to boost metabolism. In summary, metabolism plays a major role in weight loss. It's critical to comprehend how metabolism affects weight management and to adopt lifestyle modifications that can increase metabolism and promote weight loss. Achieving weight loss goals and keeping a healthy metabolism require striking a balance between overall lifestyle behaviors, physical activity, and nutrition.

Dr. Robert. R. Dixon

1.3 The link between Hormones, Metabolism, and Healthy Diet

A balanced diet, metabolism, and hormones all work together to support an individual's general health and well-being. The endocrine glands secrete hormones, which are chemical messengers that control several body processes, including metabolism. Conversely, metabolism encompasses all of the chemical processes that the body goes through to stay alive. The nutrients required for these processes to proceed effectively are supplied by a nutritious diet. The regulation of metabolism is significantly influenced by hormones. For example, the digestion of carbs, proteins, and lipids for energy is

14

regulated by hormones like insulin, glucagon, and cortisol. Insulin acts as a bridge to allow glucose to enter cells and be converted into energy, which lowers blood sugar levels. Conversely, glucagon raises blood sugar levels by encouraging the liver to produce glucose from glycogen that has been stored. Known as the "stress hormone," cortisol contributes to elevated blood sugar levels when under stress. Thyroxine (T4) and triiodothyronine (T3) are the thyroid hormones that control the body's metabolism. They accelerate the body's metabolism by raising the rate at which it uses energy. Unbalanced levels of these hormones might result in weariness, weight gain, and other health problems. Leptin, a hormone released by fat cells, is another significant hormone that influences metabolism. Through its ability to tell the brain when the body has received enough food, leptin helps control appetite and energy expenditure. Overindulgence and weight gain may result from an imbalance in leptin levels. A balanced hormone and metabolism are maintained in large part by eating nutritious food. The body gets the vital elements and vitamins needed for hormone production and metabolism by eating a wide range of fruits, vegetables, complete grains, and lean meats. A diet heavy in processed foods added sweets, and bad fats can cause metabolic slowdown and hormone abnormalities. An increased protein intake is another way to speed up metabolism. Since digesting protein uses more energy, the body expends more energy overall, resulting in a quicker metabolism. Furthermore, eating foods high in omega-3 fatty acids, which are present in foods like avocados and salmon, can aid in enhancing metabolism and balance hormones. In addition, several foods have a reputation for enhancing metabolism and balancing hormones. For instance, magnesium aids in controlling the thyroid gland's hormone synthesis, and zinc is necessary to keep the body sensitive to insulin. A nutritious diet that provides an adequate intake of

Dr. Robert. R. Dixon

these nutrients can support a healthy metabolism and assist in preserving hormonal balance.

Dr. Robert. R. Dixon

Chapter 2:

Assessing Your Present Eating Pattern

2.1   Recognizing   Unhealthy Eating Patterns

Consistent and recurring dietary practices that have a detrimental impact on a person's physical, mental, and emotional health are referred to as unhealthy eating patterns. Eating too many unhealthy meals, not eating enough nutrient-dense foods, or adhering to rigid and fad diets are common characteristics of these habits.

To enhance one's general health and make beneficial dietary adjustments, people must be able to identify unhealthy eating behaviors. Typical indicators and manifestations of unhealthful eating habits include:

1. Meal skipping or restrictive eating practices: People who regularly eat poorly are frequently the ones who skip meals or adhere to restrictive diets. Nutrient shortages, low energy, and depressive symptoms may result from this.

2.   Frequent consumption of unhealthy foods: Consuming an excessive number of processed or unhealthy meals, such as sugary snacks, fast food, and processed meats, is a common indicator of poor eating habits. These foods can raise the risk of chronic diseases since they are frequently heavy in calories, bad fats, and added sugars.

3. Emotional eating: An unhealthy eating pattern is evident when someone turns to food as a coping method for feelings like stress, boredom, or melancholy. Overindulgence, weight gain, and a

bad connection with food can result from this behavior.

4. Yo-yo dieting: Excessive calorie restriction or fad diets that cause weight loss and gain repeatedly are indicators of unhealthy eating habits. In addition to being unsustainable, this weight-cycling cycle may be harmful to one's physical and emotional well-being.

5. Obsessive calorie counting or food tracking: Restricting food intake to particular macronutrient ratios or calorie counts regularly may be a sign of an unhealthy relationship with food. Nutrient

shortages and disturbed eating patterns may result from this approach.

6. A diet devoid of diversity: Consuming the same things all the time and avoiding a wide variety of foods, like fruits, vegetables, and whole grains, might be signs of an unhealthy eating habit. An unbalanced diet and nutrient deficits may result from this lack of diversity.

7. Experiencing guilt or shame after eating: Negative emotional reactions to food, including guilt or shame, may be signs of an

Dr. Robert. R. Dixon

unhealthy eating behavior. One's physical and mental health may suffer as a result of this vicious cycle of overeating and restriction.

To enhance general health, it is critical to identify these telltale signs and symptoms of poor eating habits and take appropriate action. Here are some pointers for ending bad habits and creating a positive connection with food:

1. Emphasize moderation and balance: Aim for moderation and balance in your diet rather than rigid restrictions or excluding particular foods. Eat a range of

nutrient-dense foods at each meal, but also permit yourself to occasionally indulge in small pleasures.

2. Pay attention to your body's signals of hunger and fullness. Eat when you're hungry and stop when you're satisfied but not stuffed. Emotional and excessive eating may be avoided in this way.

3. Give up the diet mentality: Restrictive eating practices and fad diets should be avoided because they might create harmful routines and are not long-lasting. Rather, concentrate on adopting long-term

Dr. Robert. R. Dixon

lifestyle adjustments that promote a nutritious and well-balanced diet.

2.2   Identifying   Metabolic Problems and Hormone Imbalances

The process by which our body turns food into energy is called metabolism. Our cells go through several chemical reactions to maintain life. A complicated web of interactions between hormones and enzymes that control different metabolic processes affects our body's metabolism. Metabolic issues can arise from any imbalance in the synthesis or activity of these hormones and enzymes.

Disorders known as metabolic issues impact how our body uses foods and energy. Hormonal imbalances, lifestyle decisions, environmental conditions, and genetics can all contribute to them. Adrenal insufficiency, thyroid abnormalities, obesity, and diabetes are a few prevalent metabolic issues. If these illnesses are not treated, they may have a major negative influence on our general health and result in major consequences.

Dr. Robert. R. Dixon

One of the main contributing factors to the emergence of metabolic issues is hormone imbalances. Hormones are chemical messengers that are produced by the pituitary, thyroid, adrenal, and pancreatic glands, among other organs in our body. They control mood, growth, metabolism, and other essential body processes. A disruption in the synthesis or action of these hormones can cause havoc with our body's metabolic systems and result in a host of health problems.

Insulin resistance is one of the main hormone abnormalities that cause metabolic issues. The hormone insulin, which is generated by the pancreas, is in charge of controlling blood sugar levels. Insulin resistance is a condition in which the body becomes less sensitive to insulin, which raises blood sugar levels and eventually results in diabetes. Insulin resistance is known to be significantly influenced by obesity and chronic stress.

Thyroxine and triiodothyronine are two thyroid hormones that are essential for controlling metabolism. Metabolic problems can arise from an overactive or

Dr. Robert. R. Dixon

underactive thyroid gland caused by an imbalance in these hormones. For example, an underactive thyroid (hypothyroidism) can result in weariness, weight gain, and a slow heart rate, whereas an overactive thyroid (hyperthyroidism) can produce a rapid and irregular heartbeat.

The adrenal glands also create cortisol, another hormone that is vital for controlling stress and metabolism. Prolonged stress can raise cortisol levels, which can result in weight gain, hypertension, and insulin resistance. Metabolic issues can also be caused by abnormalities in other adrenal hormones, such as aldosterone and epinephrine.

Sex hormone excess or shortage can also occasionally result in metabolic issues. For example, insulin resistance, increased fat mass, and decreased muscular mass can result from low testosterone levels in men. Conversely, women who take too much estrogen may experience hormonal abnormalities, metabolic malfunction, and weight gain.

Appropriate diagnosis and treatment of metabolic disorders and hormone imbalances depend on their identification. The following are some typical indications and symptoms of these conditions:

1. Weight Fluctuations: An imbalance in hormones or a metabolic issue may be the cause of an unexplained weight gain or decrease. For example, weight increase might result from an underactive thyroid, whereas weight loss can occur from an overactive thyroid.

2. Weariness: Chronic weariness and low energy can be brought on by hormonal imbalances, which can have a big influence on our day-to-day activities.

3. Mood Swings: Hormones are mostly responsible for controlling mood. Hormone imbalances can lead to melancholy, irritability, and mood swings.

4. Insomnia: Our sleep patterns can be disturbed and brought on by changes in hormone levels, especially cortisol.

5. Appetite Changes: Hormonal imbalances can have an impact on our hunger, causing us to crave foods more or less.

6. Menstrual irregularities: Hormone abnormalities, such as those caused by polycystic ovarian syndrome (PCOS), can cause women to have painful or irregular periods.

7. Recurrent Infections: Imbalances in hormones can impair immunity, leaving us more vulnerable to diseases.

Dr. Robert. R. Dixon

Healthy eating routine to balance hormone

A healthcare provider may do a variety of tests and examinations, such as blood tests, urine tests, imaging studies, and physical exams, to detect metabolic issues and hormone imbalances. These examinations can reveal any underlying medical conditions as well as the hormone and enzyme levels in our bodies.

The underlying cause and severity of metabolic disorders and hormone imbalances will determine the course of treatment. Numerous lifestyle modifications, including a balanced diet, regular exercise, stress reduction, and good

Dr. Robert. R. Dixon

sleeping habits, might enhance hormonal balance and metabolic health. Medication may also be recommended in certain circumstances to control symptoms and hormone levels.

2. Pay attention to your body's signals of hunger and fullness. Eat when you're hungry and stop when you're satisfied but not stuffed. Emotional and excessive eating may be avoided in this way.

3. Give up the diet mentality: Restrictive eating practices and fad diets should be avoided because

they can create harmful routines and are not long-term solutions. Rather, concentrate on adopting long-term lifestyle adjustments that promote a nutritious and well-balanced diet.

CHAPTER 3

The science behind the 4-pound-per-day Weight Loss

3.1 The Impact of Specific Foods on Metabolism and Hormones

Hormones and metabolism are essential to our body's operation and have an impact on many areas of health, such as energy levels, controlling our weight, and general well-being. These two processes are greatly influenced by our nutrition, and some foods can help or impede them from working properly. We will talk about how some meals affect hormones and metabolism, as well as how they may affect our general health, in this extensive note.

The process by which our bodies turn food into energy is called metabolism. The way our bodies use and store energy from the food we eat is governed by several hormones and enzymes. Maintaining a healthy weight and avoiding chronic illnesses like obesity,

Dr. Robert. R. Dixon

diabetes, and heart disease depends on having a strong and functional metabolism. However, hormonal balance is necessary for our bodies to function properly. Hormones control mood, reproduction, growth, development, and metabolism.

Our hormones and metabolism are significantly influenced by the food we eat. While some foods can slow down metabolism and upset hormone levels, others can speed up metabolism and balance hormones. Let's examine the effects of particular foods on hormones and metabolism.

1. Foods high in protein: Not only is protein vital for metabolism, but it is also necessary for the development and repair of bodily structures. A hormone called glucagon is produced more when protein is consumed, and this hormone encourages the body to break down stored fat for energy. Moreover, it promotes the growth of lean muscle mass, which raises the body's metabolic rate. Lean meats, seafood, eggs, dairy products, legumes, nuts, and seeds are among the foods high in protein.

2. Healthy fats: Despite what the general public may think, healthy fats are essential for our bodies to function properly and can even positively influence hormones and metabolism. Healthy fats found in foods like avocado, fatty fish, nuts, seeds, and olive oil can help regulate hormones, boost metabolism, and induce satiety.

3. Whole grains: Rich in complex carbs that the body can convert to glucose for energy, whole grains are a great source of these nutrients. Additionally, they include fiber, which helps reduce blood sugar increases by slowing down the release of glucose into the system. Eating whole grains can aid in the regulation of hormones that are essential for blood sugar regulation and metabolism, such as insulin and cortisol.

Dr. Robert. R. Dixon

4. Vegetables and fruits: Vegetables and fruits are important sources of vitamins, minerals, and antioxidants, which are required for a healthy metabolism and hormone balance. Magnesium is especially abundant in leafy green vegetables. Magnesium is required for more than 300 metabolic events in the body, including metabolism.

5. Herbs and spices: In addition to giving our food flavor, herbs and spices have other health advantages. Certain spices, such as ginger, turmeric, and chili peppers, have ingredients that help increase the body's metabolism and decrease inflammation. Antioxidants, which are abundant in herbs like basil, oregano, and rosemary, can help balance hormones and enhance general health.

Conversely, certain meals may negatively affect hormones and metabolism. These consist of:

1. Processed and sugary foods: Items with little to no nutritional value, such as white bread, pastries, cookies, and sugary drinks, can boost blood sugar levels and result in weight gain and insulin resistance. They may also interfere with the body's capacity to control metabolism and upset the balance of hormones.

2. Trans fats: Tran's fats are frequently included in fried and processed meals and have been connected to a higher risk of obesity, insulin resistance, and heart disease. They may also cause disruptions in metabolism by interfering with the synthesis of hormones.

3. Alcohol: While moderate alcohol use may offer some health advantages, excessive alcohol use can alter metabolism, interfere with hormone balance, and raise the risk of obesity and chronic illnesses.

3.2 Establishing Your Body's Ideal Hormone Environment

The body uses hormones as chemical messengers to control several functions, including growth, metabolism, and reproduction. The body performs at its best and can stay healthy when these hormones are in balance. On the other hand, a range of health problems might result from a hormone imbalance.

Changing your lifestyle and establishing a healthy habit to support hormonal balance are important steps towards creating your body's ideal hormone environment. The following are important things to think about when attempting to create the optimal hormone environment in your body:

1. Nutrition & Diet

Hormone levels are significantly influenced by what you consume. The body needs a balanced, nutrient-rich diet to remain in its ideal hormonal equilibrium. Hormonal balance can be enhanced by avoiding processed and sugary foods and consuming a range of nutritious foods, including fruits, vegetables, lean meats, and healthy fats. Hormone-balancing characteristics have been found in certain foods, such as avocados, salmon, and cruciferous vegetables (broccoli, cauliflower, and Brussels sprouts).

2. Workout

Remaining physically active is essential to preserving hormonal equilibrium. Exercise has been shown to lower stress, elevate mood, and control hormone production. Research has indicated that engaging in moderate-to-intense physical activities, like strength training and cardiovascular exercises, can positively impact and balance hormone levels. On the other hand, overtraining or excessive activity might have the opposite effect and upset the hormonal balance.

3. Sufficient Rest

Sustaining an ideal hormone balance requires getting enough good sleep. The stress hormone cortisol might rise as a result of sleep deprivation, upsetting other hormone levels in the body. To help your body correctly regulate hormone levels, try to get 7–9 hours of sleep per night.

4. Handling Tension

One of the main causes of the body's hormone abnormalities is stress. Our bodies release the stress hormone cortisol when we are under stress, which can interfere with other hormone synthesis and balance. Discover healthy coping mechanisms for your stress, such as mindfulness exercises, physical activity, or fun hobbies.

Prevent Toxins

Every day, the food we consume, the items we use, and the air we breathe expose us to toxins. The endocrine system, which is in charge of generating and controlling hormones, may be disturbed by these poisons. Hormonal balance can be preserved by limiting exposure to pollutants by consuming natural and organic goods, staying away from packaged and processed meals, and leading an eco-friendly lifestyle.

6. Examine Addendums

Supplementing your diet may occasionally assist in preserving hormonal balance. To find out which supplements are best for you, speak with a medical expert because some may have negative

Dr. Robert. R. Dixon

effects or interfere with specific drugs.

7. Frequent Examinations

Seeing your doctor regularly is essential to detecting and treating any hormone imbalances early on. In addition to offering helpful advice regarding hormone levels, they may suggest dietary adjustments or, if necessary, medicinal interventions.

Determining the optimal hormone environment for your body is crucial for preserving health and enhancing general well-being. Healthy behaviors and good lifestyle modifications can help you maintain balanced hormone levels and avoid several health problems. Recall that if you have any questions regarding your hormones or notice any signs of an imbalance, you should speak with a medical expert.

3.3 How to Increase Your Metabolic Rate to Lose Weight Quickly

Our body uses metabolism to turn food into energy for a variety of internal processes. Even while at rest, a higher metabolism indicates that your body is burning more calories, whereas a slower metabolism indicates that it is burning

Dr. Robert. R. Dixon

fewer calories. Because of this, having a faster metabolic rate may help you lose weight since it burns calories more effectively. Here are some strategies for raising your metabolic rate to hasten weight loss:

> 1. Increase your muscle mass: Your metabolic rate will rise in proportion to your muscle mass since muscles need more energy to maintain than fat. Strength training activities can help you gain muscle and increase your metabolism. Include them in your workout regimen.

2. Maintain proper hydration: Several body processes, including metabolism, depend on adequate water consumption. Drinking enough water may also help you feel full and avoid overindulging, both of which can promote weight reduction.

3. Consume enough protein: Building and mending muscular tissue depend on protein. Additionally, proteins have a larger thermic impact than fats or carbs, which means that when digesting and processing proteins, your body expends more calories.

Dr. Robert. R. Dixon

4. Avoid skipping meals: When your body attempts to preserve energy, skipping meals might cause your metabolism to slow down. Consume well-balanced meals regularly to maintain an active metabolism all day.

5. Include high-intensity exercises: Even after your workout is over, high-intensity interval training (HIIT) may increase your metabolism. Short bursts of intensive exertion are interspersed with rest intervals throughout this kind of workout.

Dr. Robert. R. Dixon

6. Make sure you get enough good sleep. Sleep deprivation may mess with your hormones, especially the ones that control hunger and metabolism. To maintain the health of your metabolism, try to get between seven and nine hours of good sleep per night.

7. Steer clear of crash diets: Extreme calorie restriction might cause your body to enter "starvation mode" in an attempt to save energy, which can slow down your metabolism. Rather than focusing on drastic diets, make lasting, healthful lifestyle adjustments.

Healthy eating routine to balance hormone

Adopting these lifestyle modifications to raise your metabolic rate will help you lose weight and improve your general health. But it's crucial to keep in mind that each person has a unique metabolism and that losing weight is a difficult process with many moving parts. Speak with a healthcare provider to develop a customized strategy that works for you.

Dr. Robert. R. Dixon

CHAPTER 4

A Healthy Dietary Plan

4.1 Realizing the Significance of Macronutrients

Our bodies need a lot of macronutrients to operate correctly. They are vital nutrients. They consist of lipids, proteins, and carbs. Every one of these macronutrients is essential to preserving our general health and well-being.

Healthy eating routine to balance hormone

First of all, our body uses carbs as its primary energy source. They are converted into glucose, which our cells require for a variety of processes including organ, brain, and muscle function. Deficiency in carbs may cause drowsiness, lethargy, and trouble focusing.

Conversely, proteins serve as the building blocks of our bodies. They are necessary for hormone and enzyme production, muscle growth and repair, and the health of the skin, hair, and nails. A low protein diet may cause the immune system to become weaker, muscles to

Dr. Robert. R. Dixon

atrophy, and wounds to heal slowly.

Despite being demonized in popular culture, fats are essential for human health. They give off energy, assist in the synthesis of hormones, cushion and protect organs, and facilitate the absorption of fat-soluble vitamins. But it's crucial to restrict your consumption of harmful trans fats and eat the appropriate kinds of fats, such as unsaturated and omega-3 fatty acids.

Acknowledging the importance of macronutrients entails being aware of their functions and choosing our foods wisely. Appropriate quantities of all three macronutrients should be ingested since they are essential to our general health. Our demands for macronutrients are best met by eating a balanced diet rich in a range of complete, nutrient-dense foods.

Furthermore, some populations—such as athletes, expectant mothers, and developing children—need a sufficient intake of macronutrients. Because of their greater energy requirements and development, certain groups can need more of some micronutrients.

Macronutrients are necessary for our bodies to operate correctly, and appreciating their importance entails understanding the critical functions they play and making sure our diets are well-rounded and balanced enough to suit our demands. By being aware of the significance of macronutrients, we may enhance our general health and well-being by choosing better, more educated diets.

4.2 Planning Nutritious and Balanced Meals

To stay healthy and stave off sickness, meal planning is essential. Make sure your meals are balanced and rich in nutrients. A healthy meal is made up of a variety of food types that provide the body with the vital nutrition and energy it needs. A meal is considered balanced if it has the proper amounts of fats, proteins, carbs, vitamins, and minerals. When creating a meal plan, it's important to take age, gender, degree of physical activity, and any unique dietary requirements into account.

The essential measures to take into account while organizing a wholesome and well-balanced dinner are as follows:

1. Establish calorie needs: The first step in creating a healthy and balanced meal is figuring out how many calories a person requires each day. This may be achieved by taking into account variables such as height, weight, gender, age, and amount of daily physical activity. This will give you a ballpark idea of how many calories you'll need to keep your weight in check.

2. Opt for whole foods: Naturally high in nutrients, whole foods are unrefined, unprocessed meals. Fruits, vegetables, whole grains, legumes, nuts, and seeds are a few of them. These foods are a vital component of a healthy, well-balanced diet since they are abundant in fiber, vitamins, minerals, and phytochemicals.

3. Eat a range of meals: Eating a range of foods guarantees that the body receives all the nutrients that it needs. The nutrients that each food category offers vary, therefore it's best to include a range of meals from each to assist in meeting the body's nutritional requirements.

4. Be mindful of portion sizes: A healthy, well-balanced meal requires careful attention to quantity management. Eating the proper quantity of food is crucial to avoiding undereating and overeating. In terms of portion sizes, nutritional balance is also crucial. A portion of vegetables should be the size of your fist, but a portion of meat should be around the size of a deck of cards.

5. Add lean protein: Protein is necessary for both supplying energy and for the construction and repair of tissues. A healthy diet must include lean protein sources including beans, tofu, chicken, turkey, and fish in each meal.

Dr. Robert. R. Dixon

6. Cut down on added sweets and bad fats: Trans and saturated fats raise the risk of heart disease, thus they should be kept to a minimum in a balanced diet. Likewise, while additional sugars contribute extra calories with little nutritional benefit, they should be consumed in moderation. Alternatively, meals may include natural sugars from fruits and honey as well as healthy fats like unsaturated fats.

7. Take dietary limitations and allergies into consideration: It's important to take into account any dietary restrictions or allergies that

Dr. Robert. R. Dixon

people may have while preparing a healthy, balanced meal. A person with a dairy allergy, for instance, must stay away from dairy products and look for other sources of calcium and vitamin D, such as fortified plant-based milk or leafy greens.

8. Sip plenty of water: Staying healthy requires consuming enough water. It is advised to drink eight glasses or more of water each day. Water facilitates waste elimination from the body, nutrition transfer, and digestion.

9. Engage in mindful eating: Mindful eating entails focusing our whole attention on the flavor, texture, and aroma of the food we consume. This makes it easier for people to pay attention to their bodies' signals of hunger and fullness and prevent overeating or under eating.

A healthy and balanced diet may also be ensured by meal planning and preparation ahead of time, in addition to the previously listed methods. This entails planning a weekly menu, buying the essential supplies at the grocery store, and preparing meals in advance. Time may be saved, and maintaining a balanced diet can be made simpler.

Organizing wholesome, well-balanced meals is essential to preserving excellent health. It lowers the chance of developing chronic illnesses and aids in fulfilling the body's nutritional requirements. A balanced and healthful diet may be ensured by people by adhering to the above-listed procedures.

4.3 Including Foods That Balance Hormones in Your Daily Diet

Hormones are essential for controlling several body processes, such as mood, metabolism, and reproductive health. Stress, malnutrition, and certain medical conditions are just a few of the things that may easily cause an imbalance in these chemical messengers. Fortunately, maintaining a healthy hormone balance and avoiding associated health problems may be achieved by eating foods that balance hormones in your regular diet.

Nuts, seeds, and avocados are among the major dietary groups high in healthy fats that may help regulate hormones. In addition to being necessary for the body's synthesis of hormones, these fats may aid in lowering inflammation, which in turn helps balance hormone levels.

Hormone balance may also be supported by eating foods high in fiber, such as fruits, vegetables, and whole grains. Fiber supports the good gut flora that is involved in hormone metabolism and helps control insulin levels.

Additionally, include fermented foods may provide helpful microorganisms that help with hormone synthesis and balancing, such as yogurt, kimchi, and sauerkraut.

Traditional medicine has also used several herbs and spices, including cinnamon, ginger, and turmeric, to control hormone imbalances and regulate hormone levels.

Additionally, since processed and sugary meals may raise blood sugar levels and interfere with hormone balance, it's critical to minimize or stay away from them. Eating foods rich in quality protein, such as fish, lentils, and lean meats, may also aid in the regulation of hormones related to metabolism and the promotion of satiety.

Eating a range of whole, nutrient-dense meals may help regulate hormones and enhance general health when included in a regular diet. Before making big dietary changes for hormonal balance, it is always advised to speak with a

Dr. Robert. R. Dixon

healthcare provider, particularly if you have any underlying medical concerns.

CHAPTER 5

Typical Meal Plans for Boosting Metabolism and Hormone Balance

5.1 Ideas for Breakfast Meals

1. Avocado bread with Poached Eggs: This easy and healthful dish

Dr. Robert. R. Dixon

consists of mashed avocado, poached eggs, and a dash of salt and pepper on top of whole grain bread.

2. Breakfast Burritos: Put scrambled eggs, black beans, cheese, and any vegetables of you're choosing into tortillas. For an added kick, add some spicy sauce or salsa.

3. Greek Yogurt Parfait: For a tasty and protein-rich breakfast, top Greek yogurt with granola, fresh berries, and a honey drizzle.

Dr. Robert. R. Dixon

4. Homemade Breakfast Sandwich: For a quick and satisfying on-the-go breakfast, toast an English muffin and top it with cheese, bacon, or ham.

5. Veggie Egg Muffins: For a nutritious and portable breakfast alternative, whisk together eggs, cheese, and chopped veggies in a muffin pan. Bake.

6. Oatmeal with Fruit and Nuts: To increase the nutrition and taste of your oatmeal, add some sliced fruit and nuts.

7. Breakfast Quesadillas: These delectable and simple breakfast options are loaded with cheese, scrambled eggs, and your choice of vegetables.

8. Smoothie Bowl: To make a thick and nourishing smoothie bowl, blend your preferred fruits, Greek yogurt, and a small handful of spinach. For more crunch and taste, sprinkle granola and extra fruit over top.

9. Breakfast Tacos: Top tiny tortillas with cheese, bacon, or sausage, and scrambled eggs for a hearty breakfast. For a great and substantial dinner, serve with avocado and salsa.

10. Zucchini Fritters: For a tasty and inventive twist on hash browns, grate some zucchini, combine it with flour and eggs, and pan-fry. Accompany with a side order of scrambled eggs or your preferred morning meal.

5.2 Ideas for Lunch Meals

1. Create Your Salad Bar: Arrange a selection of raw greens, veggies, hard-boiled eggs, tofu, and grilled chicken, along with a choice of dressings. Let each guest assemble a customized, healthful salad using their components.

2. Make Your Wraps: Serve a variety of tortilla wraps, dips (like guacamole or hummus), and toppings (such as shredded cheese, deli meats, and roasted veggies). Enable each person to put together their wrap for an enjoyable and adaptable meal.

3. Baked Potato Bar: Arrange a platter of toppings, including cheddar, bacon, sour cream, broccoli, and chives, then bake a few potatoes in the oven. Everyone may add toppings to their potato to make it a substantial and satisfying lunch meal.

4. Sushi Rolls: Assemble cooked shrimp, avocado, cucumber, and cream cheese into a batch of handmade sushi rolls. Chop them into little pieces to make a tasty and convenient lunch alternative.

5. Quinoa Bowls: Prepare the quinoa per the directions on the box and arrange different toppings like chopped avocado, grilled chicken, black beans, and roasted veggies. Allow each person to assemble a quinoa bowl using a combination of their preferred ingredients.

6. Soup and Sandwich Combo: Enjoy a mouthwatering sandwich with a warm cup of soup. Choose healthier options like an avocado and turkey wrap or a grilled chicken and vegetable panini.

7. Homemade Pizza: For individual-sized pizzas, use whole-wheat pita bread or flatbread as the crust. Before putting the pizzas in the oven, lay out a variety of toppings and let everyone construct their own.

8. Omelette Bar: Arrange a selection of ingredients for omelets, including ham, cheese, herbs, and sautéed veggies.

Assign someone to prepare the omelets upon request so that you have a filling, hot lunch choice.

9. Rice or Noodle Bowls: To create individualized bowls, start with cooked rice or noodles. Arrange a variety of veggies, sauces, and proteins (such as tofu, chicken, or shrimp) so that guests may mix and match.

10. Mediterranean Spread: Arrange a platter of foods with a Mediterranean flair, including olives, falafel, hummus, and tabbouleh. For a nice and wholesome lunch, have everyone make their own pita pockets filled with anything they choose.

5.3 Ideas for Dinner Meals

It might be difficult to come up with supper menu ideas, particularly when you're pressed for time or lack certain components. However, you can easily prepare tasty, healthful, and reasonably priced meals for your family with a little forethought and imagination. These pointers and suggestions may assist you in organizing your supper menu:

1. Begin with your favorite ingredients: Consider which ingredients your family and you appreciate the most, and then begin there. This will guarantee that everyone will be enthused about the dinner in addition to making meal preparation easy for you.

2. Use a variety of cooking techniques: Keeping your meals interesting requires variety. Try varying you're cooking techniques rather than sticking to one for every meal. To get varying textures and tastes, you may cook your food on a grill, roast, bake, stir fry, or even slowly cook it.

3. Make use of the leftovers: Avoid throwing away your leftovers. You may turn them into a whole other dish. For instance, you can use leftover chicken to create a tasty stir-fry or toss it into a salad for a light lunch.

4. Theme nights: Give each night of the week a distinct theme. This may be a night for soup, spaghetti, tacos, etc. This will save you time and effort since you will already have a rough notion of what you will be constructing.

5. Meal prep: Set aside some time on the weekend to prepare some of your components in advance, including veggies, grains, and meats. You'll find it simpler to prepare a fast and healthful meal over the week as a result.

6. Try out new dishes: Don't be scared to experiment with taste combinations and try out new meals. Cooking periodicals, food blogs, and cookbooks are good sources of inspiration. You never know, maybe you'll find a new dish that you love.

7. Make use of seasonal ingredients: Incorporate seasonal, fresh food into your dishes. They are not only more tasty but also easier to get and less expensive. It's also a great way to help out your local farmers.

8. Include plant-based meals: Meals without meat are economical as well as healthful. You may want to rotate your dinners to include a few vegetarian or vegan options. Start with easy recipes like falafel wraps, lentil soup, and stir-fried vegetables.

9. Accept one-pot and sheet pan meals: These dinners are great for hectic weeknights since they're simple to make and require little cleanup. All of your ingredients may be combined and cooked in one pot or on a sheet pan.

10. Don't be scared to keep things simple: Not every dinner has to be elaborate. The simplest meals may often be the most tasty. A substantial and simple supper choice may be a loaded salad, baked potato bar, or create-your-own taco night.

In conclusion, there are many different places to get inspiration for supper recipes. Some possibilities include your favorite foods, cooking techniques, leftovers, and even your sense of adventure. You may effortlessly prepare delectable and hassle-free meals for your family by keeping these suggestions in mind. Cheers to cooking!

5.4 Snack Recommendations

In between meals, snacks may be a tasty and fulfilling method to reduce hunger. Nonetheless, it's critical to choose palatable and nourishing snacks. The following suggestions for snacks might be a wonderful complement to your routine:

1. Fresh fruits and veggies: Packed with fiber, vitamins, and minerals, fruits and vegetables are nature's ideal snack. They're a delightful and nutritious alternative since they come in a range of flavors.

2. Nuts and seeds: Rich in protein and good fats, nuts and seeds are a terrific food. They provide a quick, filling snack that will keep you feeling energetic and full.

Dr. Robert. R. Dixon

3. Yogurt: A tasty and nourishing snack is a cup of yogurt. It has a lot of probiotics, which strengthen the immune system and aid in digestion.

4. Hummus and whole grain crackers: This combo is a delicious and substantial snack. As a strong source of plant-based protein, hummus is also packed with fiber from whole grains.

5. Dark chocolate: Dark chocolate is a fantastic choice for anyone who has a sweet taste. Antioxidants, which are abundant in it, provide a host of health advantages.

Always pay attention to your body's hunger and fullness cues and choose foods that will satiate your appetites without depriving you of necessary nutrients. Maintaining a healthy diet and general well-being may be facilitated by eating in moderation and with awareness. Compose a brief memo "Snack Suggestions."

In between meals, snacks may be a tasty and fulfilling method to reduce hunger. Nonetheless, it's critical to choose palatable and nourishing snacks. The following suggestions for snacks might

Dr. Robert. R. Dixon

be a wonderful complement to your routine:

1. Fresh fruits and veggies: Packed with fiber, vitamins, and minerals, fruits and vegetables are nature's ideal snack. They're a delightful and nutritious alternative since they come in a range of flavors.

2. Nuts and seeds: Rich in protein and good fats, nuts and seeds are a terrific food. They provide a quick, filling snack that will keep you feeling energetic and full.

Dr. Robert. R. Dixon

3. Yogurt: A tasty and nourishing snack is a cup of yogurt. It has a lot of probiotics, which strengthen the immune system and aid in digestion.

4. Hummus and whole grain crackers: This combo is a delicious and substantial snack. As a strong source of plant-based protein, hummus is also packed with fiber from whole grains.

5. Dark chocolate: Dark chocolate is a fantastic choice for anyone who has a sweet taste. Antioxidants, which are abundant in it, provide a host of health advantages.

Dr. Robert. R. Dixon

Always pay attention to your body's hunger and fullness cues and choose foods that will satiate your appetites without depriving you of necessary nutrients. Maintaining a healthy diet and general well-being may be facilitated by eating in moderation and with awareness.

Chapter 6

Exercise's Contribution to Hormonal Balancing and Weight Loss

6.1 Exercises That Are Good for Hormones and Metabolism

Exercise regularly is crucial for your general health and well-being, but did you know that it may also improve your metabolism and hormones? The chemical messengers known as hormones control several biological processes, including metabolism, which is the process by which your body converts food into energy. You may raise your metabolism and assist in regulating your hormone levels by doing certain activities. We'll talk about the workouts that are beneficial for hormones and metabolism in this extensive note.

1. HIIT, or high-intensity interval training

Brief intervals of high-intensity exercise are interspersed with lower-intensity activity or rest intervals in high-intensity interval training (HIIT). It is well known that this kind of exercise increases metabolism and encourages the synthesis of growth hormone, which is essential for burning fat and gaining muscle. Moreover, high-intensity interval training (HIIT) might enhance insulin sensitivity, a crucial factor in maintaining steady blood sugar levels and delaying the onset of metabolic diseases like diabetes.

2. Strength Training

To increase muscle mass and strength, resistance training, commonly referred to as strength training, uses weights or your body weight. It has been shown that resistance exercise raises testosterone levels, a hormone crucial for metabolism and muscular building. Additionally, it enhances insulin sensitivity, which may help control blood sugar levels.

3. Asana

Yoga is a kind of exercise that combines breathing exercises, bodily postures, and meditation. Reduced levels of cortisol, the main stress hormone, have been shown. Weight gain is a possible consequence of persistently elevated cortisol levels, especially in the abdomen. Yoga may assist in regulating metabolism and fostering a healthy balance of other hormones, including insulin and thyroid hormones, by lowering cortisol levels.

4. Exercises for the Heart

Exercises that involve the heart, like swimming, cycling, or running, are crucial for maintaining a healthy metabolism. Exercise that burns calories and raises heart rate is called aerobic exercise, and it helps people lose weight. It also enhances insulin sensitivity and aids in hormone regulation, all of which support a healthy metabolism.

5. Yoga

Pilates is a low-impact workout style that emphasizes balance, flexibility, and core strength. Pilates' methodical, slow motions have the potential to increase insulin sensitivity and cortisol regulation, which may result in a more balanced hormone system.

6. Strolling

One easy and accessible kind of exercise that might improve hormones and metabolism is walking. It has been shown that brisk walking raises adiponectin levels, a hormone involved in controlling insulin sensitivity and metabolism. It's a great way to relieve stress since it also lowers cortisol levels.

7. Swinging

Not only is dancing a pleasurable and entertaining kind of physical activity, but it may also significantly improve hormones and metabolism. Serotonin, a hormone connected to mood enhancement and hunger control, has been reported to rise in response to dancing. Additionally, it may aid in lowering cortisol levels, which supports a healthy hormone balance.

In summary, frequent exercise is essential for maintaining a balanced hormone system and fostering a strong metabolism. Your hormones and metabolism may benefit from a variety of activities, among which the workouts listed above are just a few. Before beginning any new fitness program, it is important to speak with a healthcare provider, particularly if you have any underlying medical issues. You may optimize your health and well-being by supporting your hormones and metabolism with a well-rounded workout regimen, patience, and consistency.

6.2 Establishing a Successful Workout Program

Achieving your fitness objectives requires starting an effective exercise regimen. It entails putting together an organized, customized strategy that works for your requirements, objectives, and skills. An effective exercise regimen may help you gain muscular mass, increase your level of flexibility and endurance, and improve your mental health.

The following are the essential components of an effective exercise regimen:

1. Establish attainable goals: Identifying your fitness objectives is the first step in creating an effective exercise program. Whether you want to improve your general health and fitness, gain muscle, or lose weight, you need to be clear about what you want to accomplish. Throughout your exercise journey, you may maintain focus and motivation by setting clear and attainable objectives.

Dr. Robert. R. Dixon

2. Speak with an expert: To assist you in creating a successful exercise regimen, you must speak with a fitness expert, such as a personal trainer or a certified fitness coach. They may evaluate how fit you are now, talk with you about your objectives, and provide professional advice on the kinds of exercises you should do, how long to do them for, and how hard to do them.

3. Select the appropriate exercise: There are many different kinds of workouts, including functional training, strength training, cardio, and flexibility training. To create a well-rounded fitness regimen, include these activities in your

training schedule. Selecting workouts that you love and that are appropriate for your fitness level and objectives is very important.

4. Make an exercise schedule: The secret to any fitness program is consistency. Make a weekly plan that will enable you to exercise three or four times a week at the very least. Additionally, you may switch up your exercise routines to prevent overtraining and maintain interest in your activities. To help your body heal and prevent injuries, be sure to include rest days into your schedule.

5. Begin slowly and build up your exercise intensity gradually. It might be tempting to push yourself too hard while beginning a new exercise regimen, but doing so can result in burnout and injury. It's crucial to begin slowly and build up to longer and more intense exercises as your body adjusts. This will keep you encouraged to keep going on your fitness path and help avoid accidents.

6. Include a healthy diet: A fitness journey cannot be successful with only exercise. Maintaining a nutritious and well-balanced diet is essential to sustaining your exercise and promoting

106

muscle repair. To get a customized food plan that meets your fitness objectives, speak with a nutritionist.

7. Monitor your progress: A good exercise regimen requires regular monitoring of your progress. It enables you to assess your progress and determine what changes are necessary to keep advancing toward your objectives. You may use fitness apps, measurements, or images to keep track of your progress.

8. Remain responsible and motivated: It's common to go through ups and downs while trying to get healthy. Join a

fitness club, locate a workout partner, or acknowledge little accomplishments along the road to keep yourself motivated. You can remain on track and make your fitness program successful by holding yourself responsible and acknowledging your accomplishments.

In conclusion, patience, consistency, and perseverance are necessary for creating a good exercise regimen. It's critical to concentrate on your unique requirements, make reasonable objectives, and get expert advice. You may attain your fitness objectives and sustain a healthy lifestyle with the appropriate strategy, frame of mind, and work.

Dr. Robert. R. Dixon

Chapter 7

Additional Lifestyle Factors for Weight Loss and Hormone Balance

7.1 Stress Reduction Methods

Life will always include stress, which may originate from several things, including relationships, employment, money problems, and personal obligations. It may hurt one's bodily and emotional well-being if ignored. Finding efficient ways to reduce stress is thus crucial for maintaining general well-being. We will examine and talk about some of the most popular stress-reduction techniques in this post.

1. Exercise: It is well recognized that regular physical activity helps to relieve stress. Endorphins are endogenous substances released by the body during exercise that have anti-depressant and natural painkilling properties. Exercise may also aid with sleep quality, which is often disturbed by stress. Because it enables us to concentrate on our bodies and movements rather than our worries, it may also be a beneficial diversion. Exercise in any way may help lower stress levels, including dance, yoga, swimming, and jogging.

2. Mindfulness and Meditation:

The practice of mindfulness involves accepting things as they are, without passing judgment, and being totally present in the moment. Intentionally focusing on a certain idea, thing, or activity to reach a quiet and clear state of mind is called meditation. It has been shown that both of these methods are effective in reducing stress. They aid in lowering anxiety, enhancing emotional control, and encouraging relaxation. They also help us to let go of anxious thoughts and feelings and give us a sense of inner calm.

3. Breathing Methods: For a very long time, people have used deep breathing methods to soothe their bodies and minds. Stress may cause our breathing to become fast and shallow, which exacerbates feelings of tension and worry. We may reduce our blood pressure and heart rate by practicing deep breathing, which helps us cope with stress. Taking slow, deep breaths in through the nose and out through the mouth while concentrating on the feeling of the breath in our bodies is a basic method. When we feel overwhelmed, we can do this anytime, anyplace.

4.   Time   Management: Feeling overburdened by a lengthy list of duties or obligations may sometimes lead to stress. Thus, stress reduction depends on excellent time management. To help us keep organized and on track, this entails prioritizing chores, establishing reasonable and attainable objectives, and making a calendar. We may prevent last-minute rushing and the tension that goes along with it by practicing good time management.

5. Social Support: Reducing stress may be aided by having a solid network of friends and family. We might feel relieved and get a fresh perspective on our circumstances when we confide our issues and worries to a trusted person. In addition to being a beneficial stress diversion, spending time with loved ones and participating in fun activities together may also encourage emotions of enjoyment and relaxation.

6. Self-care: Taking good care of our physical, mental, and emotional needs is crucial to stress management. This includes obtaining enough sleep, maintaining a healthy, balanced diet, and participating in enjoyable activities. It also entails establishing limits and refusing requests when we are too busy or incapable of taking on new obligations. Taking care of ourselves may increase our resilience and sense of self-worth, which will improve our ability to cope with stress.

7. Getting Professional Assistance:

Stress may sometimes become too much for us to handle on our own. Getting expert assistance from a therapist or counselor may provide us with the skills and encouragement we need to deal with our difficulties in an efficient manner. Additionally, therapy may assist us in creating healthy coping skills by revealing the underlying problems that are causing us stress.

In summary, stress management techniques are essential for controlling the negative effects of stress on our physical and mental health. By incorporating these techniques into our everyday lives, we may reduce stress and live happier, healthier lives. Finding the method that works best for each of us personally is crucial, as is making an effort to regularly use these approaches in our everyday lives. We may get a more serene and well-rounded mental state by persevering and being committed to it.

7.2 The Value of quality Sleep

A condition of rest in which a person's physical, mental, and emotional well-being are entirely restored is referred to as quality sleep. It is a necessary component of human existence and is crucial to preserving general health and wellbeing. But in today's hectic environment, a lot of individuals often forgo getting enough sleep in favor of work, socializing, or entertainment. Due to this, sleep deprivation has become commonplace, which may be harmful to one's health and quality of life.

It is impossible to overestimate the importance of getting enough good sleep

Dr. Robert. R. Dixon

since both the body and the mind depend on it. Our bodies recover and restore themselves as we sleep. The body can manufacture the hormones required for tissue regeneration and repair, immune system bolstering, and maintaining a healthy metabolism when it gets enough good sleep. These functions are disturbed when people don't get enough good sleep, which may result in a number of health problems including reduced immune systems, impaired cognitive function, and a higher chance of developing chronic illnesses like diabetes and heart disease.

In addition, getting enough sleep is essential for preserving mental health and a functioning brain. Our brains assimilate information from the day and combine memories when we sleep. Additionally, the brain filters out irrelevant information when we sleep, which enhances our ability to make decisions and solve problems. Memory loss, cognitive impairment, and difficulty concentrating have all been related to little sleep. Additionally, it may exacerbate mental health conditions including anxiety, sadness, and mood swings.

The standard of our sleep has an impact on our mental health and general state of mind as well. Serotonin, sometimes referred to as the "happy hormone," is released by our body when we get enough rest and sleep. This helps control our emotions and mood. Conversely, a lack of sleep may lead to mood fluctuations, irritation, and even melancholy. Prolonged sleep deprivation may exacerbate stress and make it difficult to handle day-to-day difficulties.

Moreover, keeping a healthy weight is greatly dependent on getting enough good sleep. Hormones that control appetite may be upset by sleep deprivation, which increases the desire for unhealthy, high-calorie meals. Additionally, it may slow down metabolism, which makes weight loss challenging. Chronic sleep deprivation has been connected to obesity and weight increase, which may lead to a number of health problems including diabetes and heart disease.

Not only does getting enough sleep help our bodies and minds, but it also enhances our general quality of life. A good night's sleep enables us to wake up feeling rejuvenated and energised, which facilitates concentration and productivity throughout the day. Additionally, it keeps us from being exhausted or sluggish so that we may enjoy our regular activities.

In summary, the importance of getting good sleep cannot be overstated. It is a cornerstone of general wellbeing and excellent health. Maintaining a regular sleep schedule, setting up a comfortable sleeping environment, avoiding coffee and electronic device usage just before bed, and practicing relaxation methods to encourage deep, restful sleep are all crucial for getting the most out of good sleep. Making sleep a priority and obtaining enough rest are essential for leading a contented, healthy, and happy life.

7.3 Stay clear of hazardous substances and environmental influences

To safeguard the health and welfare of themselves and their communities, everyone must avoid dangerous chemicals and environmental factors. Any chemical or factor that has the potential to endanger human health or the environment is considered a hazardous substance. These include radiation, noise, chemicals, contaminants in the air and water, and other hazardous items.

Environmental factors and exposure to dangerous chemicals may have detrimental effects on human health as well as the ecosystem. It may result in respiratory troubles, reproductive difficulties, acute or chronic diseases, and in extreme circumstances, even death. Additionally, it has the potential to upset the equilibrium of different ecosystems and cause ecological harm.

It is essential to understand the possible sources of environmental risks and dangerous chemicals to avoid them. They are present in both commonplace goods like insecticides, cleaning agents, and personal hygiene products as well as commercial processes like production and shipping. As a result, it's critical to educate oneself about potentially hazardous materials and their impacts on our environment.

Following the safety instructions and carefully reading product labels are two ways to reduce exposure to potentially harmful chemicals. Additionally, it's critical to properly dispose of any hazardous items at waste disposal facilities, including paint, batteries, and electrical devices. By doing this, the materials are kept out of landfills and away from environmental pollution.

Furthermore, whether handling or being near dangerous items, use care and adopt the appropriate safety measures. This entails using safety equipment, according to safety procedures, and getting expert help when handling hazardous materials.It's critical to recognize and address environmental effects that have the potential to negatively impact the ecosystem. This may include using fewer single-use plastics, using less energy, and appropriately disposing of garbage. Reducing the detrimental impacts of noise pollution may also be accomplished by being aware of how it affects wildlife and human health.

Dr. Robert. R. Dixon

Additionally, it is critical for people to support and campaign for laws and procedures that lessen the use of dangerous drugs and other environmental impacts. This might include helping businesses and goods that emphasize environmentally friendly operations and getting involved in neighborhood projects like beach clean-ups and tree planting campaigns.

In conclusion, protecting human health and the environment requires avoiding potentially harmful chemicals and environmental factors. A community may become safer and healthier for present and future generations if people

127

Dr. Robert. R. Dixon

are aware of possible risks, take the appropriate safety measures, and promote eco-friendly activities.

CHAPTER 8

Monitoring Your Development

8.1 Tracking Hormone Levels and Weight Loss

Since many individuals are seeking efficient strategies to control their weight and enhance their general health and well-being, tracking hormone levels and weight reduction has gained popularity in recent years. Hormones are an important component in weight reduction since they regulate several body functions, such as hunger and metabolism.

Several hormones, such as insulin, leptin, ghrelin, and cortisol, are very important when it comes to losing weight. Insulin controls blood sugar levels and converts excess glucose into fat. Often referred to as the "satiety hormone," leptin controls hunger and energy expenditure. Known as the "hunger hormone," ghrelin increases appetite and encourages the accumulation of fat. Finally, if levels of cortisol are raised for extended periods, this "stress hormone" may lead to weight gain.

People may have a better understanding of the relationship between their hormones and their weight reduction journey by monitoring their hormone levels. People may maximize their weight reduction efforts by making educated judgments regarding their food, exercise routine, and way of life by keeping an eye on their hormone levels.

Insulin is a crucial hormone to monitor while trying to lose weight. Weight loss may be impeded by insulin resistance, a condition brought on by an excess of insulin in the body. People may do an oral glucose tolerance test or a fasting blood sugar test to monitor their insulin levels. These tests may assist in determining if insulin sensitivity is a problem that needs to be addressed and whether insulin levels are within a healthy range.

Blood tests may also be used to monitor leptin levels. Elevated levels of leptin might be an indication of leptin resistance, a condition in which the body fails to react to the hormone's cues to decrease hunger and boost energy expenditure. Leptin level monitoring may assist people in modifying their food and way of life to maintain leptin function and aid in weight reduction.

Saliva or blood tests may be used to monitor ghrelin levels. These tests may assist in determining if elevated levels of ghrelin are the cause of increased hunger and weight gain. People may modify their diets and lifestyles to aid in weight reduction by being aware of their ghrelin levels.

Monitoring cortisol levels is crucial for controlling weight loss. Reduced muscle mass and a rise in belly fat are two effects of high cortisol levels. The most common methods for measuring this hormone are blood or saliva tests. People may see any underlying pressures that could be causing them to gain weight and make the required

Dr. Robert. R. Dixon

lifestyle adjustments by keeping an eye on their cortisol levels.

Monitoring hormone levels is just a small portion of the weight reduction process. Working with a healthcare provider is crucial to correctly interpreting and comprehending the test findings. In addition, while attempting to control hormone levels and encourage weight reduction, other elements including nutrition, exercise, and sleep should be taken into account.

Finally, monitoring hormone levels and weight loss may help with weight reduction attempts and provide insightful information about a person's general health. People may maximize their weight reduction journey and enhance their general well-being by learning the function hormones play in weight loss and making the required modifications. It's critical to collaborate with a healthcare provider to accurately assess hormone levels and create a customized management strategy. People may attain and maintain a healthy weight with the appropriate strategy and lifestyle modifications.

8.2 Modifying the Meal Plan for the Best Outcomes

Making a meal plan that works for your objectives and lifestyle may be a very customized process. To get the greatest results for your health and fitness, you may sometimes need to make adjustments to your diet plan. Whether your objective is to grow muscle, reduce weight, or enhance your general health, changing your diet plan may help you get there.

The following advice will help you adjust your diet plan to get the greatest results:

Speak with a professional: It's crucial to speak with a qualified dietitian or other healthcare provider before making any modifications to your food plan. They can give you tailored advice according to your requirements and objectives.

2. Make little adjustments: In an attempt to see results quickly, it might be tempting to make significant modifications to your eating plan. Instead, it's critical to implement little, progressive adjustments. This lowers your chance of feeling overburdened or deprived and enables your body to adjust gradually.

3. Pay attention to balance: When making changes to your meal plan, remember to concentrate on arranging your food in a balanced manner. This entails consuming a range of foods from every dietary category, including fruits, vegetables, lean proteins, complex carbs,

and healthy fats, to make sure your body is receiving all the vital elements it requires.

4. Pay attention to your body: Since each individual's physique is unique, what suits one person may not suit you. Observe how your body reacts to various meals and modify your diet as necessary. This might include changing the amount of food you eat, avoiding certain items that could make you feel bloated or uncomfortable, or experimenting with new foods to bring diversity and nutrients to your diet.

5. Meal prep for success: Planning your meals will make it simpler for you to follow through on your schedule. To ensure you have wholesome alternatives on hand when you need them, set aside some time each week to plan and prepare your meals.

6. Be flexible: Your diet plan may need to adjust as your body and your exercise objectives do. To keep things interesting, try different dishes and recipes, and don't be afraid to make alterations as required.

In conclusion, you may get the optimum results for your fitness and health objectives by making adjustments to

139

Dr. Robert. R. Dixon

your diet plan. Always remember to prepare your meals, get advice from a specialist, make little adjustments, concentrate on balance, pay attention to your body, and be adaptable. These pointers can help you design a customized food plan that suits your needs and objectives.

Chapter 9

Overcoming Obstacles and Sustaining a Balanced Diet

9.1 Handling Emotional Eating and Cravings

Cravings and emotional eating are widespread behaviors that many people find difficult to break. Emotional eating is the act of consuming food based on feelings other than actual hunger. Contrarily, cravings are strong inclinations for a certain kind of food, frequently bad options.

These behaviors can have detrimental effects on one's physical and mental health, including emotional discomfort, weight gain, and dietary inadequacies. Consequently, it's critical to comprehend and acquire useful techniques for managing emotional eating and cravings. We'll talk about a few methods and approaches in this article that can assist people in breaking these bad behaviors and fostering a positive connection with food.

1. Maintain a food journal: Monitoring your intake of food will assist you in recognizing trends and situations that lead to emotional eating and cravings. Additionally, it might help you become more aware of your eating patterns and the foods you consume.

2. Recognize and control your emotions: Stress, boredom, loneliness, and melancholy are a few examples of emotions that can lead to emotional eating and cravings. Instead of turning to food as a coping strategy, people might learn to recognize and control these feelings.

3. Engage in mindful eating: This entails eating in the current moment while paying close attention to your food preferences, feelings, and physical experiences.

4. Look for substitute coping mechanisms: Seek substitute methods for handling emotions other than eating.

Dr. Robert. R. Dixon

This can involve things like taking a walk, reading a book, or having a conversation with a buddy. People can manage their emotions without overeating if they can find a healthy way to express them.

5. Fill up on nutritious options: Having wholesome snacks on hand might assist people in choosing better foods during cravings. Having easily accessible, wholesome snacks like fruits, veggies, and nuts on hand might help people satiate their hunger without going off course with their diet.

6. Steer clear of tight diets: Strict dietary guidelines and extreme diets can frequently cause severe cravings and

Dr. Robert. R. Dixon

binge eating. To prevent feeling deprived and inciting emotional eating, food must be done in a sustainable and balanced manner.

7. Engage in stress-relieving activities: Emotional eating and cravings can result from high levels of stress. People who practice stress-relieving techniques like yoga, meditation, or deep breathing are better able to control their emotions and resist the want to overeat.

8. Get Help: People who are having trouble with emotional eating and cravings may find it helpful to get help from a therapist or support group. These specialists can assist people in addressing underlying psychological

problems and creating useful eating behavior management plans.

9.2 Practical and Social Ways to Travel and Eat Out

Experiences like traveling and dining out may be thrilling and delightful, offering people the chance to meet people from other backgrounds and learn about new cultures and cuisines. Traveling and dining out have practical and social benefits in addition to recreational and leisure ones, and they can have a big impact on a person's personal and professional lives. Easy Ways to Grab Takeout:

1. Business Dinners: In the professional world, networking and forming relationships are greatly aided by attending business dinners. It enables people to get to know their clients or coworkers better and talk business in a more casual and laid-back atmosphere.

2. Social Get-Togethers: Having dinner together with loved ones is a wonderful opportunity to catch up and mingle. It can be an enjoyable and laid-back way to commemorate milestones like holidays, anniversaries, and birthdays.

3. Networking Events: Meeting new people, exchanging ideas, and establishing business contacts can all be

accomplished by going to networking events that offer food and drinks.

4. Traveling for Food: A few people go on trips expressly to sample new foods and discover various cuisines. Well-known culinary hotspots like Thailand, Japan, and Italy draw lots of tourists who want to savor the local cuisine.

5. Trying Local Cuisine: It's a requirement to sample the local cuisine when traveling, whether for business or pleasure. It makes it possible to engage with the culture through food

Social Dining Options:

1. Date Nights: One of the most common romantic activities for couples is going out to eat. It offers a unique and private space to spend quality time and make memories with your significant other.

2. Brunch with Friends: Combining breakfast and lunch, brunch has grown in popularity as a get-together activity for friends. It's a fun and easy way to catch up on the weekends while indulging in delectable cuisine and beverages.

Dr. Robert. R. Dixon

3. Potluck Parties: At a potluck party, everyone brings a dish to share with the group. It's an enjoyable and engaging opportunity to meet up with friends or coworkers and check out new foods.

4. Food Festivals: Food festivals are occasions where a range of regional and foreign cuisines are served, along with live music, acts, and other forms of entertainment. They offer an excellent opportunity to sample and discover a variety of cuisines at one location.

In conclusion, dining out and traveling have a variety of social and practical benefits that can improve a person's quality of life.

9.3 Establishing a Helpful Network

Building relationships with individuals or groups that share similar interests and goals is a crucial part of developing a helpful network for both personal and professional growth. Examples of such individuals or groups include friends, colleagues, mentors, coaches, and other professionals who share similar goals and interests. These networks can offer a variety of benefits, including access to resources, information, and referrals, as well as emotional support and encouragement. To create a helpful network, you must actively seek out and engage with people who can enhance your life. You can do this by attending networking events, joining professional organizations, or interacting with members of your industry on social media.

It takes time and effort to establish a solid and useful network. It necessitates having a sincere interest in other people and their job, being willing to help out when needed, and being engaged in both. Sustaining and fostering these relationships is crucial in order to guarantee their sustained expansion and efficacy.

Your ability to succeed both personally and professionally can be substantially enhanced by having a supportive network that offers opportunities, insights, and viewpoints. It is a useful tool that can support you as you overcome obstacles, accomplish your objectives, and keep an optimistic outlook.

Conclusion

In summary, improving your metabolism can have a big influence on your efforts to lose weight. You can lose up to 4 pounds a day and reach your weight loss objectives more quickly by

153
Dr. Robert. R. Dixon

comprehending and treating the underlying reason of a slow metabolism. Maintaining a healthy weight, getting regular exercise, and controlling stress can all help you burn fat more quickly. Keep in mind that losing weight is a process, and long-term success depends on maintaining a healthy metabolism. You'll see improvements in your physical and mental health as soon as you begin putting these adjustments into practice. Your metabolism may be healed and you can become a healthier, happier version of yourself with perseverance and dedication.